RESETTING THE BODY

A SIMPLE PLAN FOR WEIGHT LOSS FOR OPTIMUM HEALTH

MORRISON ROBERTS

TABLE OF CONTENT

INTRODUCTION

When starting a health journey, the most important thing to remember is to be patient with yourself because your body needs time to physically adjust to the changes in your diet as well as maintain this new healthy habit. According to research, it can take up to 21 days to form a new habit.

If you've been feeling tired, bloated, or just out of sorts lately, summer is a great time to reset your body. It may appear to be a daunting task — adulting is difficult enough without having to alter your daily routine — but there are numerous ways to give your body a fresh start that do not involve extreme diets (such as drinking only lemon water for days on end) or intense workouts. Rest assured that none of these suggestions involve deprivation.

CHAPTER 1

SOME WAYS TO KEEP YOU HEALTHTY

Actually, one of the most effective ways to restart your body, according to Tiye Massey, Director of Content at Clean, a 21-day detox program developed by one NYC-based Dr. Junger, is to simply eat better, rather than eat less. When I asked Massey for advice on how to give your body a fresh start, she said that the majority of it had to do with diet. "Everyone can benefit from eating more antioxidant-rich fruits and vegetables." "Antioxidants can help us look and feel better by preventing cell damage caused by free radicals, which we are all exposed to on a daily basis," Massey tells Bustle. "Jumping and even dancing can help with lymphatic function, and it only takes a few minutes."

Here's everything else I learned about how to reset your system without becoming hungover or exhausted like a gym rat.

Consume More Water

Maybe you're one of those Super Organized People who drinks several liters of water every day. Congratulations, if that's you! Keep doing what you're doing, you responsible human. If, on the other hand, you (like me) don't drink enough water, increasing your water consumption is one of the simplest ways to give your body a reboot."Start with your body weight in pounds and divide that number in half," suggests Massey. The result is the minimum amount of water in ounces we recommend drinking every day." So, if you weigh 130 pounds, you should drink at least 65 ounces of water per day. If you drink coffee and alcohol on a regular basis (guilty), you should be drinking even more. "If you exercise, drink coffee, or consume alcohol, you should drink more water,"

Remove Inflammatory Foods From Your Diet Temporarily

Temporarily avoiding foods that commonly cause sensitivities and inflammation in the body, such as "wheat, dairy, eggs, nightshades, corn, soy, refined sugars, as well as certain meats, fruits, and condiments." So, if you want to reboot your system, you'll have to eliminate most of the fun foods from your diet.

Fortunately, this break from wheat bread and other delectable foods does not have to be permanent in order to be effective. Clean can also help you gradually reintroduce some of these foods back into your diet if you think you'll need it. "You don't have to give up these foods forever — after three weeks, our Wellness Coaches help guide cleansers through a reintroduction phase to customize a healthy diet moving forward," Massey says.

Spend More Time Outside

Personally, I enjoy being outside, so I spend at least an hour each day walking, reading, writing, and/or chatting in nature. Even if you don't consider yourself the "outdoorsy type," you should try to spend more time outside because nature is extremely beneficial to our health. "People who are exposed to natural scenes aren't just happier or more comfortable; the very building blocks of their physiological well-being respond positively," The Atlantic explained in a 2013 article on the subject. So, not only can spending time in nature be a lot of fun, but studies show that spending time in nature literally resets our minds and bodies. One such study from the 1980s found that patients whose windows faced brick walls rather than trees experienced more depressive symptoms and required an extra day to recover from their operations. This study also discovered that nature may have some pain-relieving properties. According to The Atlantic, "very few of the patients who looked out onto the trees required more than a single dose of strong painkillers during the middle part of their stay, whereas those facing the wall required two or even three doses."

Buy High-Quality Foods and Cook for Yourself

I understand how difficult it can be to find the time to cook. I also understand that high-quality groceries are typically so expensive that eating out may appear to be the easier and less expensive option, but all that takeout isn't doing your health any favors. "You can't really get control of your nutrition and your health until you know exactly what you're putting in your body," The Huffington Post explained last year, "and restaurants and packaged foods are all about hiding that information from you."Spend some time learning to cook a few healthy dishes. Keep in mind that eating healthy does not have to mean completely avoiding carbs and fats, because some fats are actually beneficial to our health. "We enjoy plenty of healthy fats from fish and chia seeds rich in anti-inflammatory Omega-3 fatty acids, and our Clean office is always stocked with coconut oil, which contains medium-chain fatty acids that our bodies can easily use as energy rather than storing as excess body fat," Massey tells Bustle.

Include Vegetables and Omega-3 Fatty Acids in Your Smoothies

If the thought of consuming all the fruits and vegetables your body requires for a proper nutrition overhaul makes you feel overwhelmed, toss some of that high-quality food we just discussed into a blender. According to The Huffington Post, "making healthy smoothies is a good and simple way to start incorporating fruits and vegetables" — and by healthy smoothies, they don't just mean blended fruits and sugar. Vegetables and omega-3-rich monosaturated fats (found in avocado, flaxseeds, and chia seeds) are also important components of the smoothie equation.

Exercise on a daily basis, but not excessively.

It's no secret that exercise is good for both mental and physical health, but as Bustle reported in April, it's also an effective way to detox the body. This is evidently due to the fact that exercise increases the oxygen levels in our cells, which creates the ideal conditions for full-body circulation and sweating. However, if you don't have enough protein in your system, high-intensity workouts will do more harm than good.. Schedule Sleep Time

First and foremost, let me state that not everyone has the same sleeping needs, so your definition of "enough" sleep may differ from mine. Personally, I feel best when I get about eight hours of uninterrupted sleep per night, but the National Sleep Foundation reported last year that adults aged 26-64 do not require eight hours of sleep every night, so you'll just have to figure out what works for you. That being said, regardless of your definition of "enough" sleep, being well-rested is critical if you want to give your body a fresh start.

Sleep is an important factor in stress management and weight management. In addition, getting enough sleep is beneficial to your brain. As tempting as it is to stay up until 3 a.m. with a good book or show, you must prioritize sleep. Here are some tips for falling asleep at bedtime — and if you're feeling particularly ambitious, check out these tricks for getting up earlier as well.

CHAPTER 2

HOW DO I RESET MY BODY AFTER BAD EATING?

Discover why resetting your body isn't the key to your success and what you should do instead.Have you ever eaten something you thought was "bad," then wondered, "How can I reset my body and make up for eating poorly?" As a Registered Dietitian, this is one of the most commonly heard phrases. Unfortunately, resetting or doing things to "make up for" what you ate is not advised, healthy, or likely to produce the desired results. But, if you've had this thought or taken actions to "undo" eating foods you thought were "bad," it's completely understandable.So much of the messaging surrounding food and nutrition is about being perfect all of the time, and if you aren't, you need to detox, reset, cleanse, work out twice as hard, eat less, and so on.

You may be wondering why resetting isn't the best way to handle the situation, and what you should do instead. Continue reading and we'll get right into it!

THE REASON FOR YOUR DESIRE TO "RESET" YOUR BODY

The idea of "resetting" and "making up" for eating bad foods comes from a concept known as food morality, which is the classification of foods as "good" or "bad," "right" or "wrong."In the context of dieting, "good food" is often defined as nutrient-dense foods. They are also known as "clean," "correct," "right," or "perfect." It is typically defined by those that are associated with positive health outcomes when consumed on a regular basis. Consider lean proteins, fiber-rich starchy carbohydrates, fruit, non-starchy carbohydrates, and health-promoting fats.

On the other hand, "bad food" is typically used to describe items that have little to no nutritional value or that may be associated with negative health outcomes when consumed on a regular basis. People will typically label them as "off-limits," "wrong," or "not good." We usually think of "bad foods" as things like traditional pizza, ice cream, candy, hot dogs, chips, and the like.

So, what's the problem with imbuing food with morality?

The issue with food morality is that it has the potential to snowball and complicate your relationship with food.

When we label foods as "good" or "bad," they become black and white, right and wrong, and the food we eat (or don't eat) begins to dictate how we feel.

For instance, if we make "good" decisions, we may feel proud and confident. However, when we make "bad" decisions, we may feel ashamed and guilty. This naturally leads us to try to avoid or limit food items classified as "bad."

These food rules and harsh lines of right and wrong keep us at odds with ourselves. We tell ourselves we shouldn't eat "bad" foods, but we know we really want them, so we indulge. Finally, we want to "reset" and make amends for eating "bad" foods in the first place.

Furthermore, these thoughts and behaviors are frequently disordered, resulting in an unhealthy relationship with food and your body. As a result, your physical, mental, and emotional health will suffer.

WHY IS NOT RESETTING YOUR BODY USEFUL? (PLUS, HOW IT CAN HURT YOUR HEALTH AND LONG-TERM GOALS)

"Well, Erica, certain foods aren't "good" for me and I shouldn't eat them, so what's wrong with feeling remorseful about eating them and "resetting" in response?" you may be thinking.

As innocuous as this mindset appears to be, it actually causes a great deal of damage and harm in the long run. It results in an unhealthy, unbalanced relationship with food. One in which we are either dieting and adhering to strict dietary guidelines or mindlessly overindulging to the point of discomfort. All of this contributes to feelings of food guilt, stress, and overwhelm.

This is where we can get into trouble, and the unbalanced nature of the all-or-nothing cycle begins.

If you're unfamiliar with our Balance Spectrum tool, you can download our free guide to learn more about it!

The All Or Nothing Cycle Is Caused By Resetting

When we try to "reset" to compensate for "bad" eating, we end up doing what we call "pendulum swinging" on the Balance Spectrum. We quickly progress from the enjoyment half of the Balance Spectrum to the "all-in" end of nourishment.

The "all-in" approach may imply additional restrictions on "bad" foods, calorie counting, macro counting, strict food rules, and eating schedules. All in an attempt to "compensate" for eating "bad foods."

But what happens when we spend too much time at the "all-in" end of the spectrum? We've returned to the "all-out" polarizing end of the spectrum, you guessed it. It's not a graceful, easy slide to a little more enjoyment; it's a full-on swing to instant gratification.

Consider a pendulum. If we exert too much force in one direction, the pendulum will inevitably swing harder and faster in the opposite direction. Right? People have the same experience when they eat.

The "all-in" end may manifest as binge eating, overindulgence, and a lack of control over food with little to no regard for nutrition. The cycle simply continues from here. This is the essence of the all-or-nothing cycle.

CHAPTER 3

WHAT TO DO INSTEAD OF "RESETTING" AND "COMPENSATING FOR" BAD FOOD EATING

We now know that labeling foods as "bad" and then attempting to "make up" for eating them leads to an unhealthy, negative relationship with food. It results in a continuous swing from "all-in" to "all-out" eating.

So, what should we do instead?

Take Morality out of Food

We want to get rid of morality and celebrate both ends of the Balance Spectrum. To appreciate food for what it is.We want to keep in mind that food is simply food. It's either nourishment, pleasure, or a combination of the two. There are no such things as good and bad foods.

When we can do this, we can make food choices that feel true and right to us. We are no longer obligated to "make up" for eating "bad foods." We can glide with ease across the Balance Spectrum, rather than swinging like a pendulum back and forth from one polarizing end to the other.

When making food choices, prioritize both nutrition and enjoyment.

When we don't consider food as good or bad, we can prioritize both nourishment and enjoyment. We eat in a healthy manner.

Following are some examples of balanced eating:

Eating some foods for pure pleasure
Never eat food simply because you "should" or are "supposed to."
Not feeling guilty about enjoying but not necessarily nourishing food
Eating nutritious foods because you want to
Creating meals that include both nutritious and enjoyable foods
There will be no more "cheat" days.
When on vacation and eating outside of your normal routines, you should feel guilt-free and stress-free.

HOW TO BALANCE AND EASE YOUR EATING HABITS

This is precisely what our Mindful Nutrition Method teaches. We show you how to use our Balance Spectrum on a daily basis to reflect and take intentional, mindful action that strikes the perfect balance between nourishing yourself and enjoying food.

We walk you through the process of healing your relationship with food and teaching you how to create a new relationship that allows for growth, stability, and support.

During the pandemic restrictions, many of us lost our normal daily routines. In addition to this loss, some people gave up their daily exercise routine and frequency of movement. To mitigate Covid-19 restrictions and inactivity, a new study recommends at least 30 minutes of extra light activity per day and five minutes of movement every hour throughout the day. Here are six alternative methods for resuming your daily routine, keeping your mind and body active, and keeping your career moving.

Exercise. Exercise is good medicine, according to studies, not only for the limbs and the heart, but also for the brain. One study discovered that, after a year, exercise and movement increased blood flow to the brain and even slowed the onset of dementia.Yoga hatha. Yoga, a stress-reduction technique that includes controlled breath concentration while gently stretching the body in different poses, has been shown in studies to lower cortisol levels and promote sleep when practiced consistently. The 3,000-year-old tradition has been hailed as beneficial to the body. Yoga has been shown in numerous studies to help regulate blood glucose levels, improve muscle skeletal ailments, moderate the nervous system, and regulate the cardiovascular system. The pace is steady and slow, and the poses are simple. Stretching, body poses, controlled breathing, focused attention, mental awareness, and the meditative process are all elements of Kundalini yoga that work directly on physical vitality and increased consciousness Scientific studies show that Kundalini yoga is more effective than stress education in reducing generalized anxiety disorder. As you move through poses with names like cobra, archer, or cat cow that require balance and concentration, you will be drawn away from ruminating thoughts and worries. It is possible to leave a session with a calmer mind, a lighter feeling, refreshed, and clearheaded.

Certain types of yoga have been shown in studies to increase dopamine squirts by 65%. People with chronic pain reported that hatha yoga and mindfulness meditation relieved their pain and improved their mood and functional capacity in a recent study.It has also been reported that the practice lowers blood pressure, improves blood flow, improves cognitive functioning, and improves mood. Yoga breathing and stretching forms raise GABA (gammaaminobutric acid) levels in the brain by up to 27%. GABA has been linked to decreased depression and anxiety. Yoga was found to significantly reduce stress levels in army veterans suffering from post-traumatic stress disorder after they practiced it twice a week for 10 weeks.
Mindfulness practices Mindfulness is an effective stress reliever. According to research, how you pay attention in the present moment has a direct impact on your mind and body, your thoughts and feelings, and your interpersonal relationships. Mindfulness activates the brain's social circuitry, allowing you to focus on awareness in the present moment. According to researchers, mindfulness reduces heart rate and brain wave patterns while also improving our immune system and cardiac function. Regular meditation results in less stress, fewer health problems, better relationships, and a longer life.Tai Chi. This ancient practice is a gentle form of exercise that consists of a self-paced series of slow, flowing body movements that require concentration and lead to

mind and body relaxation. Standing, you move steadily, slowly, and harmoniously from one posture to the next. Tai chi, like yoga, keeps your attention in the present moment by focusing on a set of prescribed body movements. Tai chi has been shown to improve the quality of life in people with a variety of medical conditions, including COPD. A number of studies have also found that tai chi can help people with COPD improve their respiratory function as well as their ability to walk and engage in other types of exercise. The ombination of movement, breathing, and relaxation is thought to provide benefits. Anyone can safely and gradually strengthen their heart and major muscle groups with these movements. Deep breathing exercises increase oxygen uptake, which can alleviate shortness of breath, and the meditative aspect of the practice reduces stress.

Short relaxation techniques and massage A new study finds that short, easy-to-apply relaxation techniques can activate your body's regenerative system (the parasympathetic nervous system or the rest and digest response) to counteract stress (the sympathetic nervous system or the stress response), providing a new perspective on how we can treat stress-related disease. After only 10 minutes of receiving a massage, researchers observed higher levels of psychological and physiological relaxation in people. Even 10 minutes of simple rest increased relaxation, though not to the same extent as massage. This is the first scientific evidence that short-term treatments like massage can effectively reduce stress on both a psychological and physiological level by stimulating the parasympathetic nervous system (PNS). Massage at work can also help improve general feelings of well-being and health.A study on work-site acupressure and seated massage improved workers' overall feelings of well-being. Employees who received the massage reported increased general well-being, decreased depression and anxiety symptoms, improved emotional control, and fewer sleep disturbances. Overall, the study discovered that employees who received massage maintained their job satisfaction while those who did not received massage experienced a decrease in job satisfaction.

Yoga in a Chair Yoga can recharge your batteries right at your desk, in the chair you're sitting in, as long as it has a back. Position your left hand on your right knee. Place your right arm on the chair's back. Stretch lightly while keeping your eyes open or closed. Take note of the stretch and what happens on the inside. Bring your body back to center after 60 seconds. The stretch is then reversed. Wrap your right hand around your left knee. Place your left arm on the chair's back. Stretch lightly again, this time with your eyes open or closed. Pay attention to the stretch and what happens on the inside. Bring your body back to center after 60 seconds. You can keep going if you want to.

CHAPTER 4

BETTER METHODS FOR RESETTING YOUR BODY AND MIND

For your physical and mental well-being, you must restore, rebalance, and reset your body and mind.

It's definitely time to reset your body and mind after a long vacation during the summer or holiday seasons. For your physical and mental well-being, you must restore, rebalance, and reset your body and mind. When you are laden with toxins, there is no joy. It's time to hit the reset button when you're stiff and foggy. Who wants to spend their days feeling bloated and congested?

On this page, you will find better methods for resetting your body and mind. Remember that you don't have to do them all, but seven days of your favorites will get you back on track.

Resetting Your Body

A healthy body leads to a happier life. Taking care of your body prevents illness and stress and provides you with the energy you require. Here are some suggestions for resetting your body.

Daily Physical Activity

Everyone knows that exercise is beneficial to our bodies. From staying fit to muscle building to improving your body shape, there is something for everyone. Exercise also reduces stress, eliminates toxins, and provides energy. Begin your exercise routine by walking if you are new to in your neighborhood. If you can't handle more, start with 10 minutes and gradually increase the time. Increase the minutes gradually until you reach 30 minutes. Daily exercise will help to reset your body to a healthier state.

Drink Enough Water to Reset Your Body

Water is extremely important in maintaining our health. To keep your body hydrated, it is recommended that you drink at least 8 glasses of water per day. This, however, is dependent on your height and occupation.

Athletes who are constantly on the move will undoubtedly require more water. Drink a large glass of water after waking up in the morning and more frequently throughout the day. Water is essential for resetting your body.

It protects your tissues and muscles by acting as a lubricant for your spinal cord and joints. Water also helps to regulate your body temperature, improves blood-oxygen circulation, flushes out waste and toxins, aids in saliva production, and aids in weight loss, aids digestion, promotes glowing skin, and keeps your brain in good working order. Our bodies are 60 percent water. The more water you drink, the more your body is reset. If your water is bland, try adding a squeeze of lemon or lime. For a special treat, add some strawberries or blueberries.

Cleanse Your Body

It is beneficial to reset your body so that you can begin the next season on the right foot. We find ourselves succumbing to the temptation of eating processed foods on a regular basis. As a result, detoxing is the better option for ridding our bodies of toxins. Furthermore, detoxing should not be difficult. A 3-5 day fruit and vegetable smoothie detox can be sweet and delicious. Detoxing rids the body of toxins that can lead to disease, aids in weight loss, and boosts energy.

Get Enough Rest

It is estimated that 50-70 million Americans are sleep deprived. These figures are concerning. Your productivity is determined by how well you sleep. Better sleep is essential for brain function because it is during sleep that your brain removes waste that can lead to neurodegenerative diseases, reduces mental problems, and increases cognitive ability. When you get enough uninterrupted sleep, you'll be able to think more clearly and feel better. To be more productive the next day, it is recommended that you sleep for 7-9 hours each night.

How to Clear Your Mind

To function properly, your mind must be free of stress. You can reset your mind in this manner.

Daily Meditation is one of the most effective ways to relax your mind. Meditation reduces stress, improves attention span, and increases self-awareness. Even a 5-minute meditation session can improve your health.

You must meditate in a quiet environment. Concentrate on something that cools your mind while seated. It's normal for your mind to wander at first. Continue to concentrate and be gentle with yourself. You'll get used to it and benefit from it over time. Repeat this daily to reset your mind and keep yourself calm.

Consider the positive.

To be in a better mood, you must maintain your positive attitude. Positivity reduces stress, increases happiness, and promotes healing. You should be conscious of your thoughts. When you worry excessively, you are more likely to experience mental difficulties such as stress and anxiety. Choose to focus on what makes you happy and what you have accomplished thus far. If it's difficult for you to be happy, don't listen to your inner critic and instead seek professional help.

We live in a hectic world. This forces us to multitask. But did you know that focusing on one thing at a time helps your brain work better? Multitasking increases stress and prevents your brain from functioning optimally. When you multitask, your concentration is low, which reduces your productivity. To achieve your goal, concentrate and do one thing at a time. When you reduce stress, your mind automatically resets, leaving you with fewer worries.

CHAPTER 5

FASTING TIPS TO SAFELY 'RESET' YOUR BODY

History, culture, science, and the evolutionary adaptations of our own bodies all confirm that a well-planned fast is beneficial to our mental, emotional, physical, and spiritual well-being. For more on why fasting is such an effective "reset" for your body, read my previous blog, "Is Fasting a Reward or a Punishment for Your Body?"

Before you begin fasting on purpose, there are a few things you should know. First, prepare yourself. Fasting, for all of its benefits, can be a very uncomfortable and stressful experience if you have never done it before. But don't worry; you'll be fine despite the discomfort. Your body was built for this. The unpredictability of food availability in earlier times led to the development of bodily mechanisms to avoid malfunction when resources are scarce. We are naturally well prepared for periods when food is scarce or completely unavailable.

Who Is Not Allowed to Fast?

Take heed! Despite the fact that fasting has been practiced for a long time, not all practices are appropriate for all people. Individuals with any type of eating disorder, a BMI less than 20 or greater than 40, kidney or liver disease, a gastric ulcer, severe morbidities, alcoholism, psychosis, pregnancy, lactation, unexplained weight loss, or who take medication with diuretics or immunosuppressive premedication (except corticosteroids) should consult with an open-minded integrative healthcare professional. This list is not exhaustive, so if you suffer from any condition, you should consult with a medical provider before beginning any fasting regimen.

What You Should Know

If you are in good health or have permission from your doctor to fast, here are some guidelines to get you started. Consciously planning a fasting protocol can help you enjoy the amazing health benefits while minimizing potential negative effects. The following are some fundamental steps to take:

Increase your liquid intake in the form of pure water or herbal teas. At the same time, change your diet by increasing your raw food consumption, focusing on fruits, vegetables, nuts, and seeds. Try to avoid all flours, sugars, meats, coffee, dairy, and other processed foods.

After the first 1-2 days, begin fasting for a few hours each day. Try to plan the fast for a day when you can relax. Your body is used to a disproportionate amount of calories, and fasting may cause you to feel dizzy, light-headed, and nauseous if you are overworked. Simply take it easy.

For first-timers, aim for 2 to 6 hours without eating, beginning when you wake up. You can also do a liquid fast by drinking juices or distilled water with Himalayan salt. Because of their high enzyme counts, I recommend starting with papaya, apple, or pineapple juice mixed with spirulina or chlorella. This variation will be less shocking.

Fasting first thing in the morning is ideal. This is the time when the body prepares for the next day by eliminating the debris that accumulated during the night (remember maintenance and repair?). If you have trouble getting out of bed in the morning for any reason, you can try the fast from 5 p.m. until the next morning, eating light, nutrient-dense foods during the day.

If you choose to fast from 5 p.m. until the next morning, skip the cereal box the next morning. Recharge your batteries with nutrient-dense, restorative foods. A super-charged smoothie (Shake logy, anyone?) would be ideal.

Fasting for the first time is similar to learning to drive for the first time; you may feel awkward, uncomfortable, uneasy, or just plain strange. Just like driving, you'll be fasting like a pro in no time once you get used to the bumps in the road!

CHAPTER 6
CONCLUSION

Please keep in mind that fasting should be done on a regular basis. It is intended to be used on occasion, not as a means of creating another system or dogma to force the body to do something. It is intended to be done consciously and for the sake of one's health. Listen to yourself because you are the only one who knows what is best for you if you choose to do so. It should not be used to lose weight.

www.ingramcontent.com/pod-product-compliance
Lightning Source LLC
LaVergne TN
LVHW052114160826
845678LV00015B/3550

* 9 7 9 8 8 4 6 3 7 9 8 1 7 *